I AM CANCER FREE

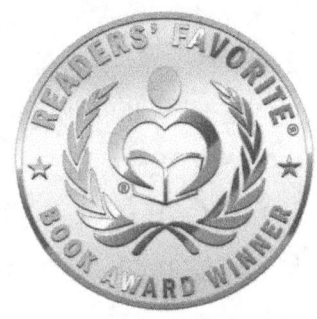

Cancer does not have to be a
Death sentence

AUTHOR: BRENDA MOHAMMED

CONTENTS

VERSE OF THE DAY 3

INTRODUCTION 4

BOOK REVIEW 6

BOAT CRUISE 9

SURGERY TURNS AWRY 13

BAD NEWS 18

MEDICAL TESTS IN MIAMI 25

HURRICANE WILMA 40

I WORE A WIG......................................43

NEW YORK 46

PRE- OPS 49

CANCER SURGERY................................53

A CROSS ON MY STOMACH.....................59

HOME FOR CHRISTMAS 62

POST SURGERY CHEMO.........................66

MIRACLE OR FALSE ALARM?...................71

NEW LEASE ON LIFE..............................75

EPILOGUE 78

TRUE VALUE OF INSURANCE 83

POEMS I WROTE 94

NEVER GIVE UP....................................101

FAVORITE HYMNS.................................103

AUTHOR'S BIOGRAPHY 112

BOOKS BY AUTHOR...............................117

VERSE OF THE DAY

"But I have spared you for a purpose
— to show you my power and to
spread my fame throughout the
earth."
–Exodus 9:16

INTRODUCTION

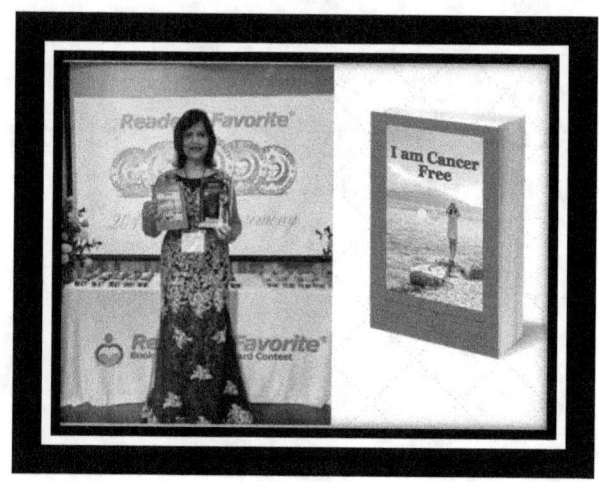

This is the true story about a woman's bout with Ovarian Cancer, a killer disease.

It has been more than sixteen years, and she is cancer free. God is alive, and he heals.

Ovarian Cancer does not have to be a death sentence. God is ever faithful and listens to those who love him.

"Trust in the Lord with all thine heart and lean not unto thine own understanding. In all thy ways acknowledge him, and he shall direct your paths." [Proverbs 3:5-6]

BOOK REVIEW

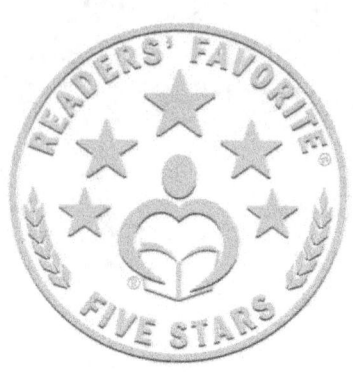

Reviewed by Mamta Madhavan for Readers' Favorite.

I Am Cancer Free by Mrs. Brenda C. Mohammed is the poignant memoir of the author's personal battle with cancer. Her faith in God and proving that ovarian cancer need not be a death sentence are what make this memoir a heartrending read.

The author's 'never say die' attitude, the decision not to give up in life, and finally being cancer-free will encourage everyone who has been diagnosed with the disease or who has suffered from cancer. The memoir recounts from the time of diagnosis the experiences the author went through during the treatment, her emotions, fears, finances, until the successful treatment of the disease. It is a courageous story of survival, faith, and strength.

The author chronicles every step of her journey methodically, without leaving anything out, making the narration very personal, honest, and palpable to readers.

The presence of God in everyone's life, a positive attitude, and the power of prayers run through the memoir. The author reiterates the fact that faith in God removes all obstacles in life.

The conversational style of writing connects well with readers, making it easy for them to understand her journey. The author has also shared the poems she wrote during that phase in her life, where she again speaks about her story, faith in the Lord, and a Higher Power.

For all those who are suffering from cancer and are battling the disease, this book is a must-read as it will give them hope, strength, and courage to fight the disease.

BOAT CRUISE

Preparing to spend a couple of months at home after a simple surgical procedure, I had no idea that I would instead spend the next several months treating a cancerous tumor.

It started on my birthday, 1st December 2004. My son's family came from Anguilla to surprise me for my birthday. My daughter-in-law had planned a surprise birthday party for me and invited all my relatives.

She had ordered lots of delicious food and drink, and everyone present had a very good time. My son was unable to travel to Trinidad, as he had to work.

After everyone had left that night, I started feeling unwell and realized that something was seriously wrong with me.

I tried to make an appointment to visit my doctor but could only get an appointment for 7th, December.

As I was about to go to bed, on the night before the appointment, one of my sisters telephoned. She told me that she received a message that my brother had passed away a few minutes ago.

It was shocking news. I had to postpone my visit to the doctor to attend the several nights of the wake and his funeral.

Finally, on December 14th, I visited the doctor for my medical problem. After she had examined me, she advised that she had to perform a minor procedure on me and I would require anesthetic.

She arranged to do the procedure at a nearby nursing home. The procedure was successful, and she allowed me to leave the nursing home the next day.

I thought that my problems were over and I started making plans for the rest of the year.

I was very successful in the Insurance business and had qualified for the Million Dollar Round Table three years in a row.

I did not intend to miss going to the Conference in New Orleans in June 2005.

The final examination for the Life Underwriting Fellowship Program was in August 2005, and I signed up for it.

My husband and I had made plans to visit my son and his family in Anguilla in May 2005.

To top it off, my friend, Jenny, and her husband, Ken, from Toronto, turned up unexpectedly for a vacation in January 2005. They planned a boat trip around the island and invited me to go along with them. My husband had to work and could not join us. One of their very good friends, who was the brother-in-law of my husband's sister, lent them his luxurious yacht and crew for a day. We had great fun that day.

The weather was fantastic, and we had the time of our lives cruising around the island of Trinidad. Now and again, the captain anchored the boat to allow the men to do fishing, while the women cheered them on each time they caught a fish.

Later that week the Insurance Company held its annual awards gala at the Trinidad Hilton Hotel in Port of Spain, and I learned that I qualified for the Million Dollar Round Table once again.

I was determined to go to New Orleans in June of that year. Life was going great, and I did not want to miss any part of it.

SURGERY TURNS AWRY

The Trinidad and Tobago Association of Insurance and Financial Advisers held its annual awards ceremony on 11th, June 2005, and I received three awards that night.

On 24th, June 2005, I left Trinidad with my Insurance friends to attend the Conference in New Orleans. Details of that trip have been described in one of my books, "Retirement is Fun: A New Chapter.

On 9th, July 2005, my son and his family came to Trinidad for the summer vacation. That same night I started experiencing a repeat of symptoms of the illness, which had commenced in December 2004.

I called my doctor to tell her that I was having recurring symptoms, and I was given an appointment to see her on 14th. July 2005. When I went to visit her, she examined me and sent me for an ultrasound and blood test. The results of both proved to be inconclusive. She advised me to do a hysterectomy as a precaution.

I deliberately tried to delay the operation, because, my son and his family, two of my sisters and their family members from abroad were coming home for the August vacation. I did not want to be in bed when they were visiting. I wanted to be around to entertain them and join in the fun. Although the doctor warned me against putting off the surgery, we settled on a date for 29th, August 2005.

On 7th, August 2005, my husband and I invited all the relatives to our home for a family gathering, and I told them about the impending surgery, which we thought, would be a simple procedure. One of my sisters said a prayer for a successful outcome.

Before my son returned to Anguilla on 11th, August, he went to the Nursing

Home to donate blood in the event that I would need it.

I wrote the LUTCF examination on 24th, August. By 28th, August 2005, all who had come from abroad had left and returned to their various homes.

My husband and I attended church the day before I went into the nursing home, and we were very impressed by the lay preacher whose message was about turning limitations into strengths. In the evening, my brother, his wife, and daughter came to visit, and my brother prayed with my husband and me for all to go well. I received several phone calls from my son and daughter abroad, sisters, in-laws, nieces and nephews, and fellow workers wishing me luck. They all assured me that the procedure was simple and that I would be okay.

My husband drove me to the Nursing Home at 6.30 am on 29th, August 2005. He said he would return before they took me to the operating theatre.

The Head Nurse assigned a room to me, and I lay in bed looking at the news on television. I watched in horror at the live coverage of Hurricane Katrina battering New Orleans. I recalled the wonderful time I had spent in New Orleans in June. It was very tragic to see the devastation that took place there because of the hurricane.

Time went by quickly. The nurses came to take me to the operating theatre at 11.30 am on a stretcher, and then lifted me on to the operating table. My husband, Rashiff, had not yet returned.

The aesthetician told me that after he injected me, I would feel sleepy. The doctor and nurses held my hands, and one nurse said not to worry that Jesus would take care of me. I believed her and felt confident that he would guide the hands of the surgeon, my doctor. I then drifted off into a deep sleep.

When I next opened my eyes, I was lying in my room in the nursing home.

I heard the door open, and my brother and his wife walked into the room.

They asked me how I was feeling. I felt like vomiting at that very instance and could not reply. Rashiff came in at the same time and handed me the bowl in which to vomit. I felt a burning where I received the cut, but no excruciating pains.

My brother said a prayer and I fell asleep. I vomited bile several times throughout the night but fell back to sleep each time without buzzing for the nurses.

I thought that the worst was over and it was just a matter of the doctor discharging me in a couple of days, and I returning home to resume my life.

BAD NEWS

The next day I felt much better, and the nurses removed all the drips and attachments from me. Later that night I attempted to walk to go to the bathroom. I called the nurse; she helped me up, and I was surprised at how well I walked. I felt that I was improving and that my doctor would discharge me the next day. On the following day, the doctor gave me news that I did not expect.

She told me that the operation was not successful and that she could not complete the procedure. There was still tissue remaining, and the left ovary, which she was unable to remove, was stuck to the colon. She said that I bled profusely when she attempted to remove it. All she could have done was to seal me up and stitch me back. In her professional opinion, it did not look good at all.

She said that she sent samples to the lab for testing and asked my husband to retrieve the results. She expressed fears that the pathology report would not reflect a good prognosis and asked if I had relatives living abroad. I told her that I had a daughter living in Miami. She kept apologizing and tried her best to prepare me for what was coming next, but I still did not take her words seriously.

The doctor discharged me from the nursing home on 1st, September 2005, and she kept apologizing and saying that she was sorry she could do nothing further for me. I began to suspect that something was terribly wrong with me and I began to question if I would die, but my husband kept reassuring me that everything would be okay. He said that we should await the results of the lab tests.

He collected the pathology results from the Lab on the afternoon of Wednesday, September 7^{th,} 2005. When he brought it home, I was too anxious to wait until the next day to take it to the doctor. I ripped it open, in spite of the fact that the pathologist addressed the letter to her. After reading it, my fears were confirmed. I had a malignant tumor on my left ovary. I had ovarian cancer. I showed it to my husband. He stood shocked.

God must have given me strength at that moment. I did not break down and cry or ranted and raved. Strangely, I felt a sudden sense of calm come over me. Thoughts of death crossed my mind but somehow, I was not fearful of death. I felt a sudden detachment from the world, and it was an incredible feeling.

Do not get me wrong. I had a great life. I had a wonderful husband, two fantastic children, three adorable grandchildren, loving siblings, a great career, and lots more for which to live. Yet, at that moment, I was prepared to die, and the world suddenly seemed insignificant to me. I felt an inexplicable joy that I was so close to meeting my Maker. It was not as if I was giving up on life. I loved my family, and I loved my life. Love for them filled my heart. I prayed silently and told God to have his way.

We took the results to my doctor the next day, and after reading it, she said that I needed to go abroad urgently, as the cancer was the type that could spread rapidly. She stated that she knew no doctor in Trinidad who could help me. She repeatedly told me to go abroad for medical help. She said it was a matter of life and death.

I was expecting this, and I remained calm. I felt a deep sense of urgency to contact my children, their spouses, my grandchildren, brothers, sisters, sisters-in-law, brothers-in-law, nieces, nephews, co-workers, and all my relatives, friends, and even my clients. I wanted to let them know that I had been diagnosed with a critical illness and to tell them how much I loved and cared for them.

When I returned home, I telephoned many of them. Many of my friends and relatives visited, and when I saw how much they loved and cared for me, I felt a strong determination to survive that ordeal. I recalled the Bible story in the

Gospel according to St. Matthew, where the woman with the issue of blood for twelve years touched the hem of Jesus' garment, and she was instantly cured of her disease. I knew that I could not physically touch Jesus, but I was sure that my prayers could touch his heart and he would heal me.

I lifted up my prayers once more to God, prayed in the name of Jesus, and asked that he healed me. I am sure that my prayer touched his heart because afterward, I felt strongly confident that he would answer my prayers. I felt deeply that He would not forsake me. I believed maybe it was a cross I had to bear, and when it was over, I would glorify God's name.

What happened from there on was none of my doing. I was recovering from a failed surgery and could not move around much. I had no energy to make plans to go abroad for further treatment.

My husband kept a steady head on and started the wheels in motion to take me to Miami to see a Cancer Specialist.

He booked our flights, and asked Michelle, my daughter in Florida, to arrange for an appointment with an oncologist. He did everything possible to expedite matters. He was an incredible pillar of support. My daughter consulted her doctor, who advised her to make an appointment for me with Dr. Leo Twiggs, an oncologist at the Sylvester Cancer Centre, University of Miami Hospital, for Wednesday, September 14th, 2005.

My husband asked me one question, "Do you want to leave for Miami on Saturday or Monday?" I replied, "Monday," because at that time, I had mixed feelings about going abroad and I wanted to delay my departure from home as long as possible.

When I realized that my husband had confirmed all plans to take me abroad, I called my bank and arranged for a significant increase in my credit card limit. The Manager granted it.

I also sought approval from my Primary Insurance Company, who was also my employers, to use my Group

Health Insurance abroad. Thank God, I had also taken out Critical Illness Insurance, and I had the strength to complete and submit my claim form before leaving Trinidad. The Insurance was payable on diagnosis of a critical illness, and it was not for a significant amount. It was in Trinidad and Tobago dollars, and after conversion to United States currency, it was minuscule, but I needed every dollar to pay the massive bills I was about to incur.

MEDICAL TESTS IN MIAMI

Our flight to Miami was scheduled to leave Trinidad at 8.00 am on Monday, September 12th, 2005. On the Sunday before we left, I invited the Pastor of my Church, Reverend Stephen Harripersad, to come to our home to give me Communion and to pray for my recovery. One of my sisters, a Church Elder, came to help serve the elements. After his prayers and after I received communion, I felt confident that I would be healed. The wife of my husband's cousin, a pastor, telephoned me and prayed for my healing over the phone. My confidence in my healing grew stronger at that point.

The night before we left, all my relatives gathered at our home to sing Hymns and say prayers for a safe trip and my recovery. They chose Hymns that made me sad, and I requested that we sing my favourite hymn, "Great is thy faithfulness," because I was confident that God would be there for me as he always had been throughout my life.

I hugged and kissed everyone and told each one that I would be home for Christmas. They were crying and looking at me in disbelief, but I was sure that God would ensure that I would be home for Christmas. My faith was firm and deeply rooted in me. The feeling of calm and peace, which came over me when I saw the lab report, which stated that I had a malignant tumour, was stronger than ever.

We had to make sudden decisions, and as crazy as they sound, we had no choice. At that time, we had three dogs that needed daily meals. Our housekeeper agreed to feed them. We gave her the house keys although we were unsure when we would be returning home. I also left enough money in the library so that she could pay herself weekly.

When we arrived at Piarco airport, for an unknown reason, the

American Airlines clerk gave us boarding passes for first-class seats, although we had booked economy seats. We were grateful, as the seats were extremely comfortable and the service was excellent. I felt that the hand of God was already moving in my life.

When we arrived at Miami airport, a wheelchair attendant escorted me in a wheelchair to Immigration. I was unable to walk the long distance having recently undergone surgery. My husband had to push the wheelchair as there was a mix-up and there were insufficient wheelchair attendants. We had no difficulty getting through Customs and Immigration. My son-in-law was at the airport to greet us, and we went to the University where my daughter worked, to take her to lunch. Our two-year-old granddaughter was in pre-school.

After lunch, my daughter returned to work, and my son-in-law took us to their home.

Later in the day, my daughter and granddaughter came home. Sophia had grown bigger and lovelier. She was just two years old and was a very playful and intelligent child. She talked a lot, hugged, kissed us, and kept calling us "gramma and grandpa." I was still weak from the surgery in Trinidad and needed to rest, so the next couple of days I rested until Wednesday, the date of my appointment with the oncologist.

On Wednesday, my son-in-law took my husband and me to the Sylvester Cancer Center at the University of Miami Hospital. I had to register on the first floor before going up to the second floor where the doctor had his office. On the second floor, we met his receptionist. She was very helpful and understanding. We had to wait a while to see the doctor, and I used that time to read the information on his card, which his receptionist gave to me.

Besides his private practice as an oncologist, he was also a Professor and Interim Chairman in the Department of Obstetrics and Gynecology at The Miller School of Medicine, University of Miami.

He was also the Associate Dean for Women's Health at the University, a Medical Director at the University of Miami Medical Center, and Clinical Service Chief at Jackson Memorial Hospital. I was very impressed with his credentials. I felt that God had chosen this doctor for me.

When it was finally my turn to see him, and he spoke to me, I was even more convinced that God had sent me to him. He was calm and very reassuring. He explained that he could not perform surgery on me soon after the first, as the body cells change after an operation, and it would be dangerous to attempt to remove anything then because the good cells may look like bad cells.

He suggested that I undergo three courses of chemotherapy treatment every three weeks to stop the cancer cells from spreading, after which he would reassess the position. First, I needed to do an MRI Scan and blood test, both of which I did the next day.

The blood test was simple, but I was pensive about doing the MRI Scan. I had heard from my nephew, who had an MRI done himself that they would place me in a tunnel for forty-five minutes and it could be claustrophobic. Both my husband and daughter went with me to the MRI Center, but only one person could have gone into the room with me. My daughter volunteered to stay with me while my husband remained in the waiting room. I tried my best to stay calm and relaxed and followed all the instructions the attendant gave me. I had to lie on a small cot, and the attendant covered me up and gave me speakers for my head so that I could listen to music on the radio. My daughter sat on a chair close to me.

Just as my nephew had described, the cot in which I was lying was lifted into the air and I was shuttled into a tunnel.

I could no longer see my daughter. I kept my eyes closed for the full forty-five minutes and listened to the music and to the attendant's instructions to breathe in and out as required. At last, it was over, and we awaited the results, which I received after a few minutes, in the form of a compact disc.

CHEMOTHERAPY

We decided to take the disc to the doctor right away, but he was not there neither was his receptionist. We went to the third floor and met another doctor who took it and promised to pass it on to Dr. Twiggs.

On Saturday, the doctor called me at the home of my daughter and son-in-law, to tell me that he had received the results of the MRI Scan and blood test, and wanted to see both my husband and me on Monday at his office. When we visited him on Monday, he confirmed his original diagnosis and suggested that I make the appointments for the chemotherapy sessions right away. Taxol and Carboplatin were the chemo drugs he recommended. He assured me that they were the best drugs available for my treatment.

The dates for the chemotherapy were 30th, September, October 21st, and November 11th, 2005.

His receptionist said that she would obtain the costs and telephone us with the figures. Later on, she took both my husband and me to view the Chemotherapy Unit. We saw patients taking chemotherapy, and they appeared quite comfortable sitting in lounge chairs and watching television. It did not seem painful or disruptive.

She told me to speak to the chemo nurse, who explained all the details of chemo and the possible side effects to both my husband and me. She advised me on what I should eat and drink. She told me that I should drink lots of water and use sunscreen if I had to go out in the sun. She said that I could get slight bone pains a couple of days after the treatment. What scared me was when she said that I would lose all of my hair from my head and other parts of my body. She said that I should buy a wig and to call her if I experienced any problems.

As my daughter had to work, my husband decided to ask for time off from his job and stay with me for the first chemotherapy session and then he would return home to go to work on October 2nd. My sister in London telephoned to say that her daughter [my niece], agreed to pay her fare from London so that she could come to Miami to stay with me for three weeks until October 20th.

Another sister in New York arranged to come on October 20th, and stay with me until October 31st, and my sister in Los Angeles decided to come on November 2nd, and leave when Rashiff returned to Miami on November 5th. I was elated that my sisters loved me so much that they wanted to spend time with me and look after me while I was ill. I praised and thanked God for such loving sisters.

I felt that I was the luckiest person in the world to have sisters, children, grandchildren, a loving spouse, and other friends and relatives, who were all willing and ready to stand with me when I needed them most.

The doctor's receptionist telephoned as she promised, to give me the costs of the chemo. She told me that it was very expensive and that I should sit down first to hear what she had to say. I was stunned on hearing the exorbitant costs. It was also a pay-first system, and I was required to pay for the treatment three days in advance.

She advised that my Group Health Insurance had no claim offices in the United States, and I could not use my Insurance Medical card. I had to use my credit card to pay the bills. Fortunately, I had requested and obtained a substantial temporary increase in the credit facility from the Credit Card Centre before leaving Trinidad.

The doctor's assistant said that they would classify me as a self-paying patient and I would receive a fair discount on all my bills. In further discussions with the doctor, he also assured us of a good discount on the medical bills.

My husband accompanied me for my first chemotherapy session on

September 30th. I was scared, as I did not know what to expect.

I had heard many horror stories about chemotherapy. I read a book where the author described her feelings after the treatment. She felt drained, felt like she was losing her mind, was delusional, lonely, emotionally drained, sick, nauseous and sleep-deprived.

From what I experienced, it was merely like IV drips, and I had no side effects, adverse reactions, or discomfort at the time. It lasted for eight hours, but I was quite comfortable in my cubicle with television and bathroom facilities. The nurses were wonderful. My husband bought lunch, and we ate in the cubicle. The day went by quickly, and my daughter came to pick us up in the afternoon.

I was amazed at how well I felt that day and the next. The chemo nurse had warned me that I would experience bone pains and they started on Sunday 2nd, October, the same day my husband left for Trinidad. They lasted for a couple of days.

On Monday when I went downstairs for breakfast, I fainted, and my daughter held on to me and called out to her husband for help. He rushed downstairs, picked me up, put me to lie on the couch, and brought me something to drink after I recovered.

My daughter called the doctor to tell him that I fainted, but he explained that I was having the typical side effects of the chemotherapy.

After a while, I felt much better. I never experienced any of the other feelings that I had read about in the book.

I never had time to be lonely as I always had a loving person with me. My granddaughter Sophia was a sweet loving and caring child and she spent lots of time with me colouring and reading stories together, when she was not at nursery school. She played with me whenever she came from school or was at home. She liked to colour, and she gave me her colouring books to colour with her. When my daughter was not at work, she would sit and watch a movie with me, or we would chat. That helped to relax me a lot.

My sister from London arrived on the scheduled date, and she was there for me in my most critical moments. Having just undergone surgery in Trinidad and then chemotherapy in Miami, I was weak, and my immune system was very low. She looked after me as a nurse would, preparing my meals and ensuring that I got nutritious foods to eat and that I took all my medication.

Sophia loved her and carried on long conversations with her. She checked on me often to see if I needed anything and tried not to leave me alone except when she needed to take a bath. When my daughter was at home, she would drive us to the mall to shop so that we would not be bored in the house all day, and so that I could get exercise.

The news of my illness spread everywhere. Friends from all over the world called and emailed me. My friends from Toronto and Virginia called often. They expressed concern and love for me and said that they remembered me in their prayers. My sister-in-law told me to speak to her sister who lived in Miami Beach as she also had cancer and recovered. I talked to her and felt very comforted.

A friend in Toronto told me to speak with her niece in Miami since she had recovered from cancer too. I did so, and she reassured me that I would recover. My sister in Trinidad emailed me every day and sent me Scripture passages. She said she sent out several prayer requests for me on the Internet and people were praying all over the world for my healing.

HURRICANE WILMA

One morning I was brushing my hair, and I saw large clumps of hair come off in the hairbrush. I looked on the bed and floor, and there were strands of hair everywhere. I showed my sister, and she helped me clean up the stray hairs. My head was almost completely bald, and I realized that I would need a wig. My daughter helped me to order two wigs from an on-line store.

The time flew quickly, and it was time for my sister to return to London and for my other sister from New York to arrive. Rose left on the morning of October 20th, and Jam came late in the afternoon. My daughter came from work and took me to the Fort Lauderdale airport to meet Jam. She brought many presents for Sophia, my daughter, and for me.

The next day was my second chemotherapy session, and Jam

accompanied me to the Sylvester Cancer Center. We looked at our favourite shows on Television, ate lunch, and passed the time while I received my treatment.

My daughter picked us up in the afternoon, and we went to a store to purchase necessities before heading home. We had heard on the news that Hurricane Wilma was heading for South Florida. We kept hoping that the hurricane would bypass Florida, but it did not.

On Sunday night, Jam and I awoke to hear the horrible howling of the wind, and when we looked out of the window, we saw the trees swaying violently. It was not a pleasant experience. It was my first experience of a hurricane and Jam's second. She was there on vacation when Andrew struck.

Trees everywhere in the street fell and then there was a power cut. We had to use torches to find our way around the house, and without the air-conditioning, the rooms were hot.

Thank God that there was no damage to the house. Only the fence around the house fell.

After the scary experience of the hurricane passed, we realized that my daughter only had an electric stove and we could not prepare any meals, so the next day her husband tried cooking meat and vegetables on the barbecue pit. It was not very tasty, but we ate the meal. There was no electricity for the next couple of days so we could not even look at television or use the home telephone. There was also no gas for cars at the gas stations, as the gas stations had no electricity to pump the gas. This went on for quite a few days.

During the week, we received the sad news that my sister-in-law's sister passed away at her home in Miami Beach. Cancer had surfaced again, and she did not survive the surgery. My sister-in-law and my niece flew from Trinidad to Miami for the funeral, which took place on Saturday.

I WORE A WIG

My daughter joined the massive line-up of cars at the gas station at 5.00 am on Friday morning to fill her car's gas tank with gas. She did not get through until 11.00 am that day. When she returned, she took Jam and me to the nearby Mall to buy black dresses for the funeral. All my hair had dropped off by then, and my wig arrived in the mail in time.

The next day we all attended the funeral at Grace's Funeral Home in Miami. I wore my wig. We were happy to see our sister-in-law and niece from Trinidad and other relatives who lived in Miami, and whom we had not seen for a long while. After the funeral, we went to the home of the deceased at Miami Beach, and we met more relatives and friends. It was nice meeting everyone although we met at such a sad event.

No one seemed to realize that I was wearing a wig.

On Sunday, my daughter took us to meet a couple of nieces and we went shopping in Aventura Mall. We spent a great day together. It was soon Monday and time for Jam to leave us. She left at 3.00 pm on Monday. Sue was due to arrive from Los Angeles on Wednesday, but I was not alone on Tuesday. My son-in-law was at home that day, and he cooked a nutritious lunch for me. It was delicious, and I enjoyed it.

Sue, who is a College Professor, came from Los Angeles as planned on Wednesday, and she too brought many gifts for my daughter, granddaughter and me. She gave me lots of nighties and a lovely, red, warm jacket with pretty embroidery.

On Saturday, my daughter dropped Sue and me to the Mall while she went to the airport with Sophia to pick up my husband who was returning to stay with me.

They met us at the mall later, and my husband went to J.C. Penney to take advantage of the big sale on gents' wear.

That night we all went to the Red Lobster Restaurant to celebrate our daughter's birthday, and we enjoyed a delicious meal. Sue left on Sunday, as my husband's bosses agreed that he could stay with me in Miami for as long as it took me to complete my treatment. I thanked God that Rashiff had such understanding bosses.

NEW YORK

The doctor's   receptionist called me on Monday 14th November to advise that the doctor scheduled me for surgery on 8th December 2005 and to do all pre-operation tests on 1st December, my birthday. Chills ran up my spine and I had scary thoughts about undergoing another operation. *Would it be successful this time or would it fail once more? What if the doctors found that they could not remove the tumour?*

I knew the surgery was necessary, and I wanted to go through with it. I left it in God's hands.

I told my husband that I needed a change of environment before the surgery and we discussed this with my sister in New York. Jam suggested that we go to her place in New York and stay for as long as we liked. We decided to go to New York and planned to return to Miami on 30th, November.

My daughter helped us to book a flight on the internet, and the following day we left for New York.

New York was freezing cold, and we wore warm gear to venture outdoors. Jam lived in the heart of Manhattan, and her workplace was next door to her well-heated apartment. She worked as a Foreign Service Executive Officer at the Trinidad and Tobago Diplomatic Center. Her posh apartment overlooked the city.

Stores lined the streets where Jam lived. They were all decked off with beautiful Christmas decorations. I knew that after I had the surgery, I could not do any shopping, so my husband and I did our Christmas shopping there. We bought Christmas gifts for friends and relatives to take back to Trinidad. Somehow, I felt that I would recover and return home for Christmas.

Jam's husband, who was retired, cooked delicious meals for us A niece and her friend came to visit us the day before Thanksgiving, and they bought us

Chinese lunch and a pecan pie. On Thanksgiving Day, my sister and her husband prepared a sumptuous meal for us.

A nephew, who was studying at Howard University in Washington, joined us for Thanksgiving Dinner. The three weeks went by very quickly, and it was time to return to Miami. We left New York to return to Miami on 30th November 2005.

PRE- OPS

We booked in at Days Inn, a hotel very close to the Sylvester Cancer Center in Miami. My daughter and granddaughter came every evening to visit us and take us out in the few days before my surgery. They took us to Bayside Shopping Mall, where I bought three more wigs in different styles and colours. By that time, I was completely bald from the chemotherapy treatments. Every hair on my body had fallen off except my eyebrows. What a sight I was!

It was difficult for me to look in the mirror and see the drastic change in my appearance, but I tried to put it out of my mind and dressed up in my wigs. Besides none of my loving friends and relatives had anything negative to say about me.

My daughter encouraged us to have fun, and she took us for a boat ride on the Island Cruise Queen, which sailed around Miami. When we returned to the shore, there were singers and entertainers everywhere, and my two-year-old granddaughter danced along to the music. It was indeed enjoyable.

Later that evening we had dinner at the Hard Rock Café. When we finished dinner and were about to leave it started raining, I felt like doing something daring, like dancing in the rain. It was something I always wanted to do and was never brave enough to do so. The doctor had warned me that if I got the flu they would not be able to give me chemotherapy. I had always tried not to get wet in the rain during my chemo sessions. I thought as I no longer needed chemo why not take the chance?

I put a plastic bag on my head and started dancing in the rain. My husband and granddaughter did the same and joined me as we waited for Michelle to get the car to take us back to the hotel. Fortunately, no one got the flu.

Soon it was my birthday. My friend in Toronto sent me beautiful flowers, which brightened up my morning. On that day, I had to go to the hospital to do all the pre-operation tests. The tests took almost the whole day, as I had to go from one building to the other to have them done.

First, I had an appointment at the anesthesiologist for 9.00 am. It was more like an interview to discuss if I had surgery before and if I had any allergies. Then I did a blood test at the Lab and an electrocardiogram at the hospital. The worst test of all was the CT scan. I had to drink two bottles of baroid, then sit, and wait for two hours before doing the scan. The Scan itself took less than fifteen minutes and was not bad. Then I had to do chest X-rays. It was about three-thirty when we got back to the hotel. I felt sick and had to rest a while.

My daughter and granddaughter came later to take us to dinner at the Cheesecake Factory in Coconut Grove to celebrate my birthday. Michelle told the waiter that it was my birthday, and after dinner, all the workers came around with a cake and candles and sang Happy

Birthday to me. It was a lovely end to a stressful day of hospital tests.

My son and his family stopped off in Miami to see me on their way to New York for a vacation, on 5th December. They surprised us and took the Days Inn Shuttle at the airport to bring them to the hotel. They spent a couple of hours with us at the hotel, and that visit filled my heart with joy. I hugged my grandchildren and played with them, as I was not sure if I would see them again.

I showed them my bald head, but it made no difference to them. They told me that they loved me and prayed every day for my recovery. We had lunch together, and they had fun trying on my wigs. We accompanied them on their return to the airport in the Days Inn Shuttle, which brought us back to the hotel.

It was a wonderful surprise to have them visit.

CANCER SURGERY

I was required to pay for the surgery a week before the scheduled date, but I had not yet received refunds from the medical claims, which I had submitted to the Insurance companies for my medical bills. Rashiff and I were getting worried because my credit card was at the maximum limit. I had received part payment from one Insurance Company for a dread disease claim. We deposited the amount to the credit card, but that was not enough to cover the card balance, which comprised of the excessive cost of the three chemotherapy sessions, lab tests, and pre-operation tests.

However, the day before the surgery, my primary insurers for the Group Medical Insurance paid a percentage of the claim, and that helped to reduce my credit card balance.

The Accountant at the hospital's administration also advised that they had agreed to lower the cost of the chemotherapy, so I had a credit surplus on my bill. I was able to pay the required sum for the surgery just in time.

8th December 2005 finally arrived. My daughter took the day off from work, and both she and my husband accompanied me to the University of Miami Hospital for 11.00 am. The doctors and nurses took me to a special room where several nurses prepared me for the surgery. My daughter and husband waited in the reception area. The aesthetician gave me an injection, and I started feeling drowsy.

At that stage, one of the Doctor's assistants explained the surgical procedure to me. She warned me about everything that could go wrong. It sounded scary and complicated, but I was too sleepy and dazed to worry. In my drowsy state, they gave me documents to sign agreeing to the surgery and confirming that I understood the risks involved. It was bad timing, but I signed the papers, as I was confident that God would be in the operating theatre guiding the doctor and his team. They allowed my daughter and my husband to come into the preparation room to see me until it was time to take me to the operating theatre. At 1.00 pm, the nurses told both of them that they should kiss me and leave. That was the last thing I had remembered before they took me into the surgical theatre, which I never saw. I must have fallen asleep while they wheeled me into the theatre.

When I awoke, I was in the recovery room. The nurses were trying to wake me. My tummy felt very sore. My husband was standing by my bed, and he told me that the doctor said that the five and a half hours surgery, although very complicated, was a complete success. My daughter came in and said the same thing while I was half-asleep. I praised and thanked God for his faithfulness and then fell asleep.

Both my daughter and husband had remained in the hospital until my surgery was completed.

They spoke to the doctor after the operation. He had explained the details of the process, and he assured them that I would be fine.

The next morning, I awoke feeling even more sore from the surgery. A nurse came and told me that she wanted me to get off the bed and sit on the chair so that they could make the bed and take me to the hospital room. With great difficulty, I was able to do so. A few minutes afterwards, a male nurse wheeled me away to the main hospital section and gave me a room. My husband was already in the room waiting for me.

Early in the morning, the doctor came to see me. He told me that the surgery was a complete success. It was a relief to hear him say that. He described the procedure of the surgery to me. He said that my colon had wrapped around the ovary and tumor, and it took quite a while to unravel and remove the ovary, tumor, and surrounding tissues.

It was a major operation, and the procedure took five and a half hours.

He said that as a precautionary measure that I should do three sessions of chemotherapy in January, February and March 2006.

His Assistant, who was also an oncologist, came to see me later in the day. He recommended that I do a chest x-ray and kidney and bladder scan that same day to ensure that everything was in working order again. A wheelchair assistant came to take me to the radiology department to do those tests. The results were normal. The doctor was pleased, and so was I.

When I returned to the hospital room, I saw my daughter and granddaughter in the room. Two-year-old Sophia was questioning the nurses as to the whereabouts of her grandma. I heard her say, "Where is my grandma? What have you done with her?" The nurses were laughing and enjoying conversing with her.

As soon as she saw me, she ran towards me, and I explained to her where I had been. She looked relieved.

A CROSS ON MY STOMACH

I went to use the bathroom in the hospital and looked at the cut on my belly. The first cut was horizontal and the second was vertical. I had a cross on my stomach. Did that mean something? For me, the cross means salvation, healing, and God's love.

The sweet singing and guitar strings of Christmas carolers filled the air. At that time, my husband, daughter, and granddaughter were visiting me. We looked out of the room and saw about one hundred women and men dressed in red and white, walking through the corridors of the hospital serenading the patients. They were entertaining, and brightened up the hospital. I certainly felt the Christmas spirit.

I had several visitors while I was in the hospital.

Many of my cousins-in-law who lived in the area came to see me. I also received several phone calls from many of my relatives and friends from all over the world who told me that they were praying for me. The nurses were very attentive and kind. I remember in particular Nurse Katherine and Nurse Andrea who took excellent care of me.

On the night before the doctor discharged me from the hospital, he told me that my hemoglobin level had dropped too low, and I needed two pints of blood. I received the blood during the night.

The next day I felt strong enough to leave the hospital, and I asked the doctor if he would discharge me. He was rather hesitant to do so, as he wanted to observe my progress a bit more. He jokingly asked if it was cheaper to stay in the hotel than in the hospital. That was indeed true! After a bit of negotiating on my part, both the Doctor and his assistant agreed that I was strong enough to leave the hospital.

A wheelchair assistant took me to the ground floor, and my husband arranged for the hotel van to pick me up and take me to the hotel.

While at the hotel, I rested a lot, as I was unable to go anywhere. I attempted to go downstairs with the elevator one day to check my email on the hotel's computer. My husband went with me. I felt sick right after checking my mail. I vomited in the elevator and corridor on my way back to my room. One of the cleaners saw what happened and she cleaned up the mess, for which I was very grateful.

HOME FOR CHRISTMAS

Dr. Leo Twiggs told me to return to the hospital to see him one week after my surgery. I kept the appointment. I told him that I wanted to be home in Trinidad for Christmas and that the only flight available was on 17th, December 2005. He examined me carefully, and stated that I was fine and fit to travel to Trinidad on 17th, December. I was overjoyed. I had told my relatives at home that I would be home for Christmas and I would be keeping my promise.

I also told him that I might decide to do the three sessions of chemotherapy in Trinidad if the drugs were available. He agreed. He said that I needed no other medication and only needed a daily multi-vitamin. My daughter and granddaughter spent the night of 16th, December with us at the hotel.

Michelle drove us to Miami International Airport on 17th, December.

Rashiff arranged for a wheelchair to take me to the departure gate in Miami International Airport. I had to sit in the wheelchair area for a very long time while Rashiff checked in, as there were long lines.

When the plane landed in Piarco airport, I cried with joy. Upon arrival, an attendant escorted me in a wheelchair to Immigration and Customs. My son, grandson, and sister were in the waiting area to greet me, and I was overjoyed to see them. It felt good to be home. It was a joyful reunion. God had answered my prayers and made it possible for me to be home for Christmas, just as I told them that I would.

The next day and the days that followed, I received several phone calls and visitors. Florabelle came every Saturday to spend the afternoon with me. Sometimes we would go shopping in the mall.

I enjoyed sitting in the Television room and watching cartoons with my four-year-old grandson, Andre.

He insisted on looking after me, and he stayed with me always and was willing to do any small chores for me.

He would get me water and juice from the refrigerator anytime I needed, even if it meant climbing to reach the top shelf. He even helped me choose my clothes and matching slippers and helped me to select a wig to wear out of the five that I had bought in Miami. He wanted his grandma to look pretty all the time despite her illness.

Ashley joined us at times. She was growing up to be such a sweet child. She loved her brother Andre, and he loved her too. We had fun together playing TV games and looking at cartoons. I felt blessed to have three grandchildren at that point, Andre, Ashley, and Sophia. They were a great source of therapy for my illness. In 2008 my fourth grandchild, George was born. He is the son of my daughter and son in law in Miami and a delightful little boy.

My nephew and niece-in-law invited all the family to spend Christmas

Day with them. We enjoyed the many delectable traditional Christmas dishes they prepared.

It was a pleasure to meet all the family there and share our experiences with one another. To me, Christmas that year had a lot more meaning than on other occasions, mainly because I felt lucky to have lived to see another Christmas Day. Another niece invited us over for lunch on the day after Boxing Day, and again we met with all the family and had a lovely evening.

POST SURGERY CHEMO

Time was flying, and I was getting nowhere with my attempts to do my chemotherapy treatments in Trinidad. My husband had spoken to an official in the Cancer Society of Trinidad and Tobago and a couple of doctors, but the drugs were not available, and I could not get an appointment to start the first treatment. I then called Dr. Leo Twiggs in Miami and arranged to do the sessions at the Sylvester Cancer Center, where they are most efficient. I made an appointment for 20[th,] January 2006. I started preparing for my trip back to Miami.

My sister, who worked in New York at that time, was on vacation from her job until 25[th.] January, and she agreed to go with me to Miami. We booked a flight for 17[th.] January so that when we arrived in Miami, I could do the blood test in time before the chemo session. The flight left on time, and landed in Miami at 12.02 pm.

Again, I required wheelchair assistance to go through Immigration and Customs. Upon arrival, my sister called my daughter on her cell phone, and she confirmed that she and my granddaughter were on the way to pick us up at the airport.

They soon arrived, and since we could not check in at the hotel until 3.00 pm, we all went to have lunch together at a restaurant.

After lunch, my sister wanted to visit some acquaintances at the Trinidad and Tobago Consulate in Brickell, and my daughter agreed to take us. We spent a couple of hours at the Consulate chatting with my sister's friends and then went to the hotel to check into our room

The next day my sister and I walked across to the Sylvester Cancer Center very early, to have my blood test done. After doing that, we went to the International Health Center to pay for the Chemotherapy and returned to the hotel to have breakfast.

We then took a taxi and went to Aventura Mall to do a little shopping.

On Thursday, we took a cab to Bayside where we walked around the shops, had lunch at Chilli's and then returned to the hotel to relax. My daughter and granddaughter came later that evening, and we went to the Cheesecake Factory for dinner. On Friday, we got up very early to go to the Sylvester Cancer Center for my Chemotherapy treatment.

The receptionist recognized me right away and called out to me. The chemo lasted seven hours, and by 2.30 pm, we were out of there.

We returned to the hotel and waited until Michelle and Sophia came. When they arrived, they took us to Village at Merrick Park. We just walked around and ate ice cream and pasta, did a little shopping, and then drove back to the hotel. Michelle and Sophia spent the night with us, and they took us to Miami International airport the next morning to get our flight back home.

We arrived in Trinidad safely. My brother and his wife invited us for lunch. We met Barry and Lyn Coker from Gloucestershire in the United Kingdom, there. Barry was the Vicar of Stroud. He told me that both he and his wife prayed for me during my illness.

My friend from Toronto telephoned me and said that her niece, who had spoken to me in Miami and reassured me that everything would work out for me and that I would recover, also died. She too had suffered a long battle with cancer. At that stage, I wondered what my fate was.

On Monday 23rd, January 2006, Rashiff called me from his office to say that he had received disturbing news. The twenty-year-old son of our very dear friends was involved in a road accident on the night of Saturday 21st, January 2006, the same day Jam and I returned from Miami. He died on the spot. It was shocking. I called up my friend who confirmed the news. I was not well enough to visit them at their home and remembered them in my prayers every night. I was determined to attend the funeral and Rashiff and I attended the cremation at Belgrove's Funeral Home on Wednesday 25th, January 2006. It was sad to see a young life depart this earth just when he was ready to accomplish so much.

He was a handsome chap. All those who made speeches spoke very highly of him. The funeral reminded me so much of one eleven years ago. The nineteen-year-old daughter of one of our friends who worked at the Bank with us died in a car accident in Toronto in 1994. It was heartbreaking.

.

MIRACLE OR FALSE ALARM?

Once again, I made plans for my second post-surgery chemotherapy in February. My husband had bought all the tickets for the second and third trips in advance. My illness was costing a fortune, but the Insurance Companies paid well on my claims. Thank God for Insurance!

I had begun to recover from the soreness of the surgery, so Rashiff and I attended church at the end of January and the first week in February. I was well enough to sit through the whole service comfortably.

On the second trip, my niece, Rhonda, went with me. When I returned home after the second chemotherapy session, I felt ill for a couple of weeks and had a constant pain in my left side.

It eased up after a couple of days. My final and third chemotherapy treatment was in February 2006. My husband and I left on Carnival Monday for Miami.

On Tuesday, we went to Quest Diagnostics Center to do my blood test and afterward we had breakfast at Au Pain in the University of Miami Compound.

We then went to Bayside, and in the afternoon, Michelle and Sophia joined us for dinner at the hotel. On Wednesday, we went to the International Health Center to make the payment for the final chemotherapy treatment. I had an appointment with my doctor for 2.45 p.m. He examined me and found that I was fine. He took a Biopsy and promised to send the results to me by electronic mail.

That evening at the hotel, I received a phone call from the doctor's receptionist who told me that I had to repeat the blood test. She said that the one I did on Tuesday showed up too many discrepancies in my blood. My white blood cell count was much too low amongst other things, and the hospital could not give me chemotherapy in that condition.

I had to do a repeat test, and if the results showed improvement, then they would give me the chemotherapy. It was very worrying for Rashiff, Michelle and me. What could have gone wrong at this end-stage of my treatment? Rashiff called his sister in Trinidad and soon the news spread.

Everyone who knew about it lifted up his or her prayers to heaven, and God started fixing the problem. The next morning Rashiff and I left early for Sylvester Cancer Center. We had breakfast in a cafeteria and then I went to repeat the blood test. The nurse told me to wait in the chemotherapy Unit until they checked it.

At 9.00 am, a nurse came and said that the results were fine and that I could proceed to take the chemotherapy. She said that apparently there was an error in the original test I took. Was it a miracle or was it a false alarm? I thanked God that once again he answered our prayers.

I finished chemotherapy at 3.30 p.m. and Rashiff, and I went back to the hotel to wait on Michelle and Sophia. When they arrived, we went for dinner at Villagio, in Village at Merrick Park. When we returned to the hotel, Rashiff said a prayer to thank God that my treatment was finally over and I got the green light to go home. He also prayed for Sophia who had the flu. As usual, both Michelle and Sophia spent the night with us and took us to the airport the next day. The flight was due to leave at 9.50 am but had to be delayed for two hours, because the tail of the plane had no power, and the mechanics had to fix it.

NEW LEASE ON LIFE

We returned to Trinidad safely on 4th. March 2006 at 4.00 pm. We had a problem getting our luggage. It was rather funny, though. A friend of Rashiff's niece brought a suitcase with a wedding dress for us to take to Trinidad. The niece was getting married in June. With the lighting in the hotel room, the bag appeared to be black. Rashiff tagged it and put it together with our red ones. At Piarco airport, we got our red suitcases. We kept waiting for the black one, but everyone else collected the black suitcases. There was a navy blue suitcase going round and round the carousel, and we suddenly found ourselves alone with the navy blue suitcase. Rashiff decided to check it, and it was the suitcase with his nametag!

I received the results of the Biopsy by e-mail as promised by my doctor. I was cancer free. It was a time to rejoice and praise God once more. When I looked back over the period of my illness, I realized that it all happened for a reason. That reason was to glorify God's name and spread the word of his healing power, love, mercy and grace. Rashiff and I held a small Thanksgiving Service with the close relatives at our home on 27[th,] May 2006. My daughter Michelle and my granddaughter Sophia came to Trinidad from Florida to attend.

I also received the results of the Insurance Examination I took before my first surgery. I passed with distinction. I even won two Insurance Industry Awards in 2005 although I had only worked for eight months in that year and had qualified again for membership in the Million Dollar Round Table. However, according to one of my friends, my most valuable award was the restoration of my health by God.

I did my quarterly medical checks in early June, and all the results showed negative for cancer.

By the middle of June, I was back to my usual self and enjoying the new lease on life that God had given to me.

I continue to do annual medical checks, and they are always negative.

Two years later, my doctor in Trinidad died of cancer. It was shocking.

EPILOGUE

WHY I WROTE THE BOOK

Almost eight years after my battle with Ovarian Cancer, I decided to write the book, "I am Cancer Free."

My thoughts were that I was still alive, although my doctor in Trinidad had given up on me eight years before when she performed a hysterectomy and could not remove the tumour. I believe that my story would help others in similar situations to get other doctors' opinions, even if it means going to another country to do so. Do not rely on the first one. My experience also proves that cancer does not have to be a death sentence.

For eight years, the feeling that I would die remained with me. Even after the doctor in Miami declared me Cancer Free after seven months of treatment and surgery, I asked him, "How long do I have?" He looked at me in the eye and told me, "Brenda, I just told you that you are cancer free. Enjoy living." He also said that I should eat lots of eggs and drink lots of water.

I wrote about what I did after each chemotherapy session. Although chemotherapy filled my body with Taxol and Carboplatin, I felt energized, wanted to go shopping, and eat in restaurants. I never lost my appetite. I could have eaten any food I wanted and I drank lots of Ensure. I loved the delectable salmon dishes at Cheese Cake Factory.

Chemotherapy sessions were on Fridays and I had no pain until Sundays, when I experienced bone pains, which the doctor told me to expect.

It has been twelve years since I am Cancer Free. The cost of the medical treatment would have been great cause for concern. The total cost was US$ 123,000.00, and that is equivalent to TT$787,200.00. How did we pay that vast sum?

Well, thank God for Insurance. I had two Critical Illness Policies and Health Insurances with two well - known Insurance Companies.

The only problem was that I had to fork out that money before the Insurance Companies reimbursed me.

Luckily, as I mentioned in an earlier chapter I had negotiated and secured a large credit limit on my credit card, and I utilized that to my advantage. I also got bonus miles on that credit card which helped me to travel to and from Miami for my last three chemotherapy sessions.

In the final analysis, Insurance paid my bills, although it was a hassle to get them to do so. I always like an Insurance advertisement I saw on Television. It goes like this. "*Insurance is a promise to pay.*" Insurance has not only helped me in my bout with cancer but in all other aspects of my life.

I must also mention the generosity of my former employers at the bank where I worked before I moved on to the

Insurance business. They sent me a cheque for a rather substantial amount to help me pay my medical bills. I was so touched that I cried when I received it.

I want to take this opportunity to acknowledge the kindness of everyone who supported me at a time when I faced my greatest challenge in life. To the family and friends of loved ones who may be going through cancer treatment, I want to leave a few suggestions.

1. Do not assume that the patient does not want visitors. A couple of friends told me that they thought that I was in too much pain and that I did not want to see them. They could not have been more wrong. I was in no pain and loved having visitors.

2. I welcomed all phone calls. Never once did I refuse a call from a well-wisher. Please call the patient whenever you can.

3. A friend of mine often sent me flowers, and another sent me mementos of Hope, Courage, and Faith. I loved

those gestures. If you can afford to send flowers or something to show that you remember them, do so.

4. I thank God that my daughter, sisters, and husband, were always around and ready to take me shopping or for dinner. Offer to take your loved one to the mall or somewhere he or she would want to visit. Family means a lot to a cancer patient. So do friends.

5. I still checked my emails every day. Send an email to say how much you care and are thinking of them.

6. Pray unceasingly. *"More things are wrought by prayer when we have faith and believe."*

Be there for your loved ones. A cancer patient would appreciate the smallest gesture.

Love conquers all.

TRUE VALUE OF INSURANCE

"If I had my way I would write the word "INSURE" over the door of every cottage and upon the blotting book of every man because I am convinced that for sacrifices that are inconceivably small, families can be insured against catastrophes which otherwise could smash them up forever. It is our duty to arrest this ghastly waste, not only of human resources, but of National Wealth and strength, which follows through the death of the breadwinner. The frail boat in which the family has embarked flounders, and the women and children are left to flounder helplessly in the dark waters of a friendless world."

The above are strong words uttered by Sir William Churchill, but they are true. Despite claims that Insurance Companies are fraudulent operations, with proper safeguards, Insurance is the best protection.

Have you made adequate financial plans for your life? Are you among the many who have disregarded the need for Insurance of any kind? Most people consider the monthly or annual premiums to be a burden on their finances. On the face of it, it can seem so, for you must pay premiums for many years. Many feel that money is being deducted from their account and no immediate benefits are received. When disaster strikes or one has passed the qualifying age to buy insurance, only then does one recognize its true value.

In this article, you will read about several examples of why Insurance is a necessity.

Is Medical and Critical Illness Insurance necessary?

In my first job at a Bank in Trinidad, my employers allowed all employees to participate in a Group Medical Plan. The employer paid the larger portion, and the employee paid one-third. If the employee or any member of his/her family obtained medical treatment, he/she was required to pay all costs and then submit a claim form to the Insurance Company.

The Insurance Company would then reimburse the employee a percentage of that claim.

When you are young, medical claims are very rare, and can never add up to the premiums you pay monthly. You are tempted to cancel the insurance and save the money you spend on premiums, especially when you have so many other bills to pay in the ordinary course of life.

Patience is the greatest virtue, and if you have patience, it always pays off in the long term.

I can give you examples from my experience, and that of others. After I had retired from the Bank, I continued to maintain my medical insurance as it was part of my retirement benefits. Fortunately, for me also, I was still fit enough and enthusiastic enough to work.

I accepted a job at an Insurance Company, and they too provided me with a medical plan, as it was compulsory for every employee to have one. I also purchased a Critical Illness Insurance Policy.

Lo and behold, I was diagnosed with Ovarian Cancer five years later!

If you have a critical illness, it can be most devastating. Not only the patient suffers, but every member of the family, as well as relatives and friends, feel the pain when a loved one is in such a situation.

My bout with cancer cost a total of US$123,000.00 and in Trinidad and Tobago Dollars that is equal to $787,200.00, which is more than three-quarters of a million dollars. This is where I say, "Thank God for Insurance!" and I mean it with all my heart.

My medical insurance combined with critical illness insurance payouts covered US$113,000.00. The rest came out of my savings.

Sixteen years hence, I am still Cancer Free.

Without those insurances, I would not have been in a position to afford overseas treatment, and may not have been here today. I know of several of my friends, who never bothered to buy Medical or Critical Illness insurance, and have even surrendered their valuable policies, and are now either lying in a coma or are dead and buried.

In another instance where **Medical Insurance** saved the day, was when my husband was involved in an accident in Miami and sustained three broken ribs. For one night of treatment, he was presented with an enormous bill for approximately US$27,000.00, which is about TT$172,800.00. It took time, but his medical insurance paid the bulk of it. The other party who caused the accident paid the rest of the bill.

To this date, both my husband and I continue to benefit from medical insurance.

Property Insurance is also necessary. In certain countries, it is not compulsory to insure your property, and therefore many people live every day in danger of losing their properties. Luckily, my husband's sister and her husband had their home insured. One hot night a mysterious fire burnt their house to the ground. They escaped with their lives. They suffered great inconvenience for a few months, as they had to make do at the home of relatives.

It was worth it when they moved back into a brand new home built with the proceeds of the Insurance claim. I know of others who suffered similar misfortune and are still awaiting help from the State. **Property Insurance** usually provides protection against the following:

Theft or vandalism

Damage by Fire or Flood

Personal Liability

Automobile Insurance provides you with protection against the loss of, or damage to your vehicle. It also protects you from liability resulting from injuries caused by your vehicle to other people or property.

I recall the time when my son crashed my brand new vehicle, which I had lent him to attend university classes. I am grateful to God that not one hair of his head was harmed in that accident. The car, however, was a complete write-off and the Insurance Company settled generously.

Owning Insurance is indeed wonderful.

I have not yet experienced the benefits of **Life Insurance** personally, but I have seen the marvel of life insurance in the life of others during my Insurance career. I have seen faces filled with grief turned into faces full of joy when they receive a cheque for Life insurance proceeds.

I quote below a definition of Life Insurance:

"*Life Insurance is a contract between you and a Life Insurance Company. It specifies that the Insurance Company will provide either a fixed sum or a periodic income to your designated beneficiaries upon your death.*"

Life Insurance can serve in many ways after your death.

1. It can replace your earned income for the benefit of your dependents.

2. It can eliminate outstanding loans, mortgages, or any other outstanding debts.

3. It can pay your funeral and other final expenses.

4. You can leave an inheritance for children or grandchildren.

I know of husbands who died unexpectedly and left their wives without the financial means to look after the children.

Their children suffered and missed gaining proper Education. I also know of those who passed on and left the proceeds of Life Insurance to their loved ones, who suffered no hardship.

Life Insurance is an expression of Love. A person who dies and leaves life insurance to a spouse is demonstrating his/her undying love for that person.

A Business can also purchase **Keyman insurance** on the life of the business owner or top executive. In the event of his premature death, proceeds of the Insurance can continue to run the company. Key man insurance provides peace of mind to business owners and shareholders because they know that the company can continue operations in the event of the loss of a key employee. If death or disability strikes, key man insurance may be the difference between the company's demise and its ultimate success.

It is now time for a word on **Retirement Planning.** Advances in health care and health maintenance have helped to increase the life expectancy of the average retiree. A longer life means that individuals and couples will experience a longer retirement period. Retirees have lots of time on their hands and love to travel. They may need big-ticket items like holiday homes and cottages.

To enjoy the lifestyle retirees crave, they cannot rely on a public pension. Insurance Companies sell registered and unregistered pension plans, which can provide tax benefits and savings for the future. All employees should start contributing to a pension plan at an early age to reap the benefits when they retire. The secret is to have more than one pension plan, so that when they mature you can have multiple sources of income, which will allow you to live the lifestyle you desire after retirement.

My advice to all who read these chapters is that if you wish to live a comfortable life now and after retirement, you should consider taking out all aspects of Insurance.

Insurance is a promise to pay. It is a necessity for all. Do not leave home without it.

POEMS I WROTE

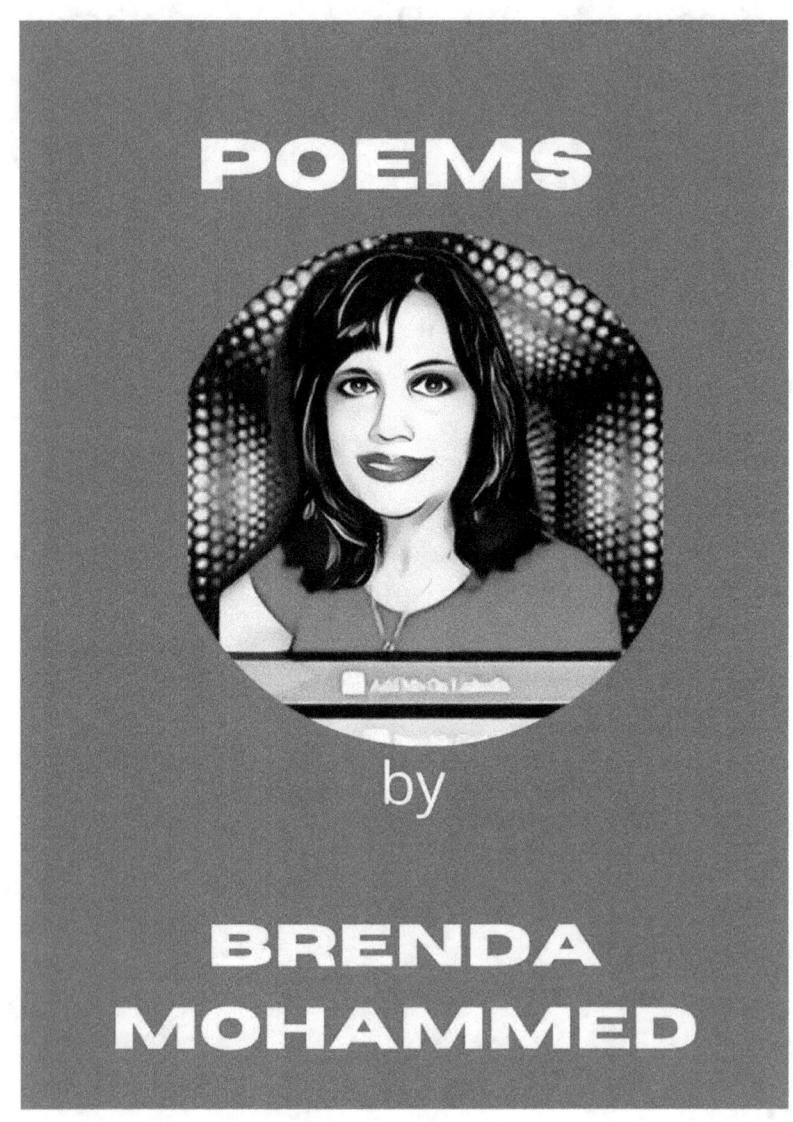

A TRUE TALE

I awoke dazed, confused, where could I be?

Suddenly recalling I just had surgery.

Hooked up to machines, nurses surrounding my bed.

I closed my eyes and covered my head.

The doctor entered, her head bowed,

She uttered that I needed to go abroad,

The surgery was incomplete, and she was sorry.

A malignant tumor was discovered in my left ovary.

My husband and I gasped in disbelief.

Fate had bestowed on me such grief.

We thought it was a simple hysterectomy.

I now needed chemotherapy and more surgery.

We immediately flew to Miami,

Where our daughter arranged for me to see

An oncologist at a cancer center;

No other doctor could have been better.

His diagnosis and treatment were very exact,

He prescribed three chemos to stop the cancer attack.

He operated and removed successfully

Every piece of the tumor that almost killed me.

I am now at home with my beloved family.

I now know how much they love me.

They were at my side as far as I recall,

My God was most faithful throughout it all.

THE HIGHER POWER

I know there is a higher power above,

He guides me and shows me much love.

The Creator's love is true

He will never disappoint you.

My thoughts and wishes line up in my head

I think of them each night I go to bed.

Like airplanes at airports lined up for flight

My wishes are granted at the Creator's delight.

I marvel at the things God has done for me.

At eight, I almost died from drowning in the sea.

My father saw my long hair floating in the water

He pulled me up before I drifted further.

At nine, an appendectomy almost took my life,

Again, God wanted me to survive.

He needed me to live to tell my story

To tell others of his mighty glory.

Later in life when cancer struck

I did not depend on sheer luck

I trusted in my Maker to heal me

Moreover, I am alive today as all can see.

I remembered the woman with the issue of blood,

Who touched Jesus' garment and obtained a flood,

Of healing power which cured her disease.

I knew that he would do the same for me.

I had no garment to touch, but I sang like a lark.

With fervent prayers, I touched his heart.

He directed my path to a doctor in Miami.

Through that doctor, he healed me.

NEVER GIVE UP

A famous writer said we are
spiritual beings

Having an earthly experience with
human feelings.

Life is not a bed of roses so we are
fighting to cope.

Trying our best to survive and
holding on to Hope.

Even if life is tough keep moving
along.

Do not let the first hurdle throw you
down.

Never ever give up there is so
much you can do.

Search for your talents what I say
is true.

Life is the sum total of the choices you make.

Do not dwell on mistakes or even heartbreak.

Believe in yourself no matter what you do.

Many of us are multitalented and so are you.

If you're fed up of life close your eyes and envision.

In a few years from now you can accomplish a mission.

Your purpose on earth is too valuable to forsake.

The choices are all there only you can make.

FAVORITE HYMNS

GREAT IS THY FAITHFULNESS

Great is thy faithfulness, O God my Father.

There is no shadow of turning with thee.

Thou changest not, thy compassions they fail not.

As thou hast been, thou forever wilt be.

Chorus

Great is thy faithfulness! Great is thy faithfulness!

Morning by Morning, new mercies I see.

All I have needed thy hand hath provided.

Great is thy faithfulness, Lord unto me!

Summer and winter, and springtime and harvest,

Sun, Moon, and stars in their courses above.

Join with all nature in manifold witness

To thy great faithfulness, mercy, and love.

Repeat Chorus

Pardon for sin and peace that endureth,

Thy dear presence to cheer and to guide.

Strength for today and bright hope for tomorrow.

Blessings all mine, with ten thousand beside!

THE LORD'S MY SHEPHERD

The Lord's my Shepherd
I'll not want
He makes me down to lie.
In pastures green, He leadeth me
The quiet waters by.

My soul, he doth restores again,
And me to walk doth make.
Within the paths of righteousness
Even for his own Name's sake.

Yea though I walk in death's
dark vale.
Yet will I fear no ill.
For Thou art with me and Thy rod
And staff my comfort still.

My table Thou hast furnished
In presence of my foes.
My head Thou dost with oil anoint,
And my cup overflows!

Goodness and mercy all my life
Shall surely follow me.
And in God's house forevermore
My dwelling place shall be.

Article in Million Dollar Round Table Magazine March/April 2007

Planning to spend a couple of months at home after a simple surgical procedure, Brenda Christobelle Mohammed had no idea that she would spend the next several months treating a cancerous tumour.

Brenda, a four-year MDRT member from Trinidad postponed a doctor recommended surgical procedure to late summer 2005 to allow her to attend the 2005 MDRT Annual Meeting as planned in June in New Orleans, Louisiana.

The day after the surgery, Brenda's doctor told her news she did not expect. The procedure had been interrupted because of what the doctor found, and she was awaiting lab results.

A few days later, Brenda was discharged, instructed to retrieve the results, and then bring them to the doctor to open. However, Brenda was too anxious to wait. "*I ripped open the envelope and was stunned to see the comments,*" she said. "*I had a malignant tumour.*"

The doctor had more bad news. The cancer cells were the type that could rapidly spread and required immediate treatment abroad.

Brenda obtained the name of a well-referred oncologist and flew to the United States to see him. "He was calm and very reassuring, explaining that he could not perform another operation so soon after the first," she said. The oncologist recommended that she do three sessions of chemotherapy to stop the cancer from spreading before he could do another surgery to remove the tumour.

When the whirlwind of the cancer diagnosis began to die down, new fear about the cost of treatment crept up on her.

She was forced to stay in the United States for several months to receive treatment.

Though she was able to stay at her daughter in Florida, the treatments were expensive at US$16,000.00 per session.

Before she left Trinidad, she thought ahead, and submitted claims for her two critical illness policies, worth US$65,000.00.

Her employers provided group medical insurance, but she had to pay upfront and submit the claims afterward.

"When the doctor's assistant called with the cost of the chemotherapy, it was very high, but luckily I had critical illness insurance and the peace of mind that I had the funds," she said.

With the second surgery, the doctor successfully removed the tumour, and the chemotherapy treatments had stopped any spreading. As a precaution, she continued chemotherapy for three months, first returning to Trinidad to celebrate Christmas with her family.

Between the chemotherapy treatments, both before and after surgery, and the surgical and hospital fees, her bout with cancer cost US$123,000.00. Her health insurance combined with critical illness insurance payouts covered $113,000.00, leaving her savings to bear the rest of the burden.

"Without those insurances, my savings and those of my husband would have been depleted completely, and we may even have had to borrow some," she said. This experience has made me more determined to tell everyone about the value of insurance. Without it, I would not have been in a position to afford overseas treatment, and be here to tell my story."

AUTHOR'S BIOGRAPHY

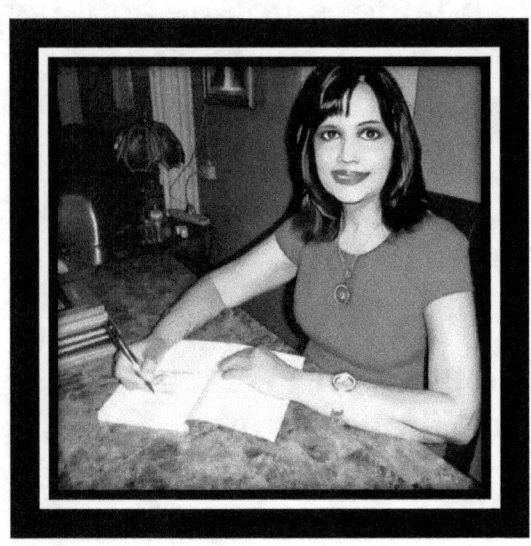

From Banker to Author, who would have imagined that a harrowing diagnosis of cancer could change your career and open up a whole new world!

Trinidadian Author Brenda C. Mohammed did not choose writing as her career. It happened by chance.

A former Bank Manager, she is a multi-genre, bestselling, and multi-award-winning author. To date, Brenda has self-published forty-six books and donates books to library and schools.

Among her publications are four anthologies and three magazines, co-authored by members of the How to Write for Success Literary Network that she founded in February 2018.

Her genres include memoirs, science fiction, romance, self-help, mystery, children's books, psychological thrillers, Christian books, poetry, and poetry anthologies.

Brenda holds a Diploma in Banking from the Institute of Bankers in London[AIB], and a Diploma in Life Underwriting from the American College, USA. [LUTCF]. She qualified for the Million Dollar Round Table, the Premier Association for Financial Professionals, [MDRT] six times in a row.

She is the Founder of the Literary Network How to Write for Success with sub-forums - Poems for Suicide Prevention, Library of How to Write for

Success, and Poems against Domestic Violence.

In May 2022, she was appointed President of Camara International Chamber of Writers and Artists Intercontinental [CIESART], for the Trinidad and Tobago office.

Her superb writing skills won her several literary awards in the USA, Peru, Kazakhstan, Seychelles, Nigeria, India, Romania, Argentina, Morocco, Philippines, Hong Kong, Indonesia, Barcelona, France, Switzerland, Italy, Indonesia, Ukraine, Sri Lanka, and the UK. She made headlines in several newspapers around the world.

Many of her books received five-star awards from Readers Favorite International, and many attained No 1 bestseller ranking.

In November 2018, she won two awards from Readers Favorite International for her science fiction book, 'Zeeka Chronicles' in the category Young Adult Thriller, and her Memoir, 'I am Cancer Free' in the category Health and Fitness.

Three of her books won gold awards in Connection EMagazine Readers' Choice Awards - Zeeka Chronicles, [2019] Stories People love, [2020] and How to Write for Success [2020]

In Sept 2021 her mystery book, Barry Holmes Mysteries, won her BEST WRITER - FANTASY Award in the CLR [Culture, Literature and Research] Awards.

Brenda is an advocate against Domestic Violence and Suicide, and together with several bestselling authors have published four Amazon No 1 best-selling anthologies for these causes: A Spark of Hope I and II, and Break the Silence I and II. Another Anthology – Peace Begins with US, will be published in April 2022.

Brenda's YouTube Channel for her Video Book Trailers, songs, and travel memories, received over 141,000 views since its inception.

BOOKS BY AUTHOR

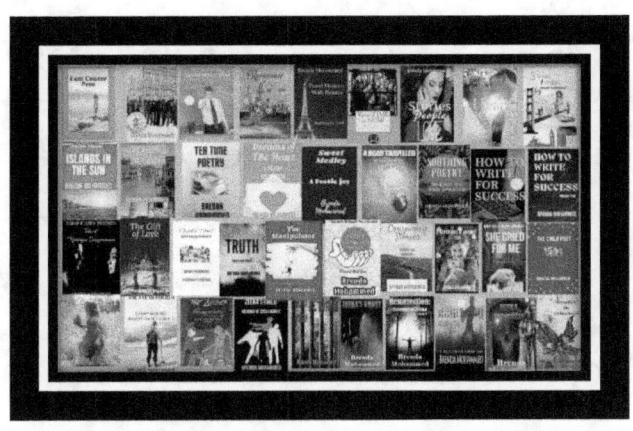

CHILDREN'S BOOKS

2014 - Adventures of Squeaky Doo– Five exciting travel Memoirs of a Teddy Bear that children love.

2017 - She Cried for Me – the heart-wrenching autobiography of a stray dog. The book is also available in Audio.

2020 -The Child Poet – A poetic Galaxy for Children, was a hot new release within hours of being published.

FICTION THRILLERS

2021 -The Manipulator: A Psychological Thriller - This thriller will have you holding on to your seat with your eyes glued to its pages.

2021 – Conspiracy Stories – Within this book, you'd find three chilling and addictive stories to awaken your mind.

MYSTERY THRILLERS

2018 - The Gift of Love: Barry Holmes Mysteries Book 1 – a crime fiction/romance.

2019 - The Axe Murderer: Barry Holmes Mysteries Book 2 – a crime fiction highlighting kidnapping for ransom.

2020 - What happened to Mary Loo: Barry Holmes Mysteries Book 3 – a suspense-filled mystery about a businesswoman who mysteriously disappeared just after the CoVid 19 lockdown.

2020 - Barry Holmes Mysteries: Tales of Mysterious Disappearances – Three mind-blowing tales of mystery.

MEMOIRS

2013 - I am Cancer Free: A Memoir – the true story of the author's miraculous recovery from cancer.

2014 - Memoirs of Dr. A. M. Khan: Journey of an Educator – gives a glimpse into life in the days of Indentureship in Trinidad and Tobago.

2014 - My Life as a Banker: A Life Worth Living – a motivational memoir of Brenda's life in the banking sector.

2014- Retirement is Fun: A new Chapter – filled with travel adventures after the author moved on from a banking career.

2014 - Travel Memoirs with Pictures: Exploring the world – a pictorial memoir of the author's travels around the world.

CHRISTIAN BOOKS

2014 - Your Time Is Now: A Time to be Born and a Time to Die – gives answers to compelling questions.

2022 – He is the One: A book for End Times. This book gives answers about eternal life.

2022 – Chosen by the Creator – It's time to wake up because these are not normal times. This book will enlighten all on God's plan for humankind. The Holy Bible has all the answers.

POETRY

2019 - Strength for the Disheartened: Motivational Poems – a collection of poems to motivate and inspire.

2019 - Dreams of the Heart: A Poetry Collection – a selection of a number of unique poems for romantic poetry lovers.

2020 - A Road Travelled: Poetry to Delight – the book features a wide range of inspirational poems on Love, Love's woes, Travel, Happiness, and effects on life during lockdown at the time of CoVid 19.

2020 - Soothing Poetry in English and Spanish - The poems are didactic, fun to read, and full of hope and insight.

2020 - Chaotic Times: Poetry Vaccine for Covid 19 published jointly with Florabelle Lutchman.

2020 – Sweet Medley: A Poetic Joy contains a medley of poems by Author Brenda Mohammed on varied subjects of life, love, and nature.

2021 – Just for You: Poetic Flowers – contains poems of love, childhood, and sundry thoughts, as well as Love poems.

2021 – Truth - Both poetry and prose within this book are about truth.

2021 – Teatime Poetry - A collection of different styles of poetry.

2021 – Treasured Memories – A collection of travel poems that will motivate readers to achieve more in life.

2021 – Islands in the Sun – Poetic verses about Trinidad and Tobago, the author's homeland.

ROMANCE

2014 - Stories People Love– Six exciting short stories of crime, adventure, and love. The stories are very alluring.

2014 - Heart-Warming Tales– Six thrilling and suspenseful tales of Crime, Love, and Unhappy Marriages.

2019 - Stories that Intrigue - a romance novel, contains the love story of Sam and Julia.

SCIENCE FICTION

2016 - Zeeka and the Zombies: Revenge of Zeeka Book 1 –the first book in a spine-chilling science fiction series and a No 1 best seller.

2016 - Zeeka's Child: Revenge of Zeeka Book 2– Mystery surrounds the birth of Zeeka's Child.

2016 - Zeeka Returns: Revenge of Zeeka Book 3– Zeeka decides his fate.

2016 - Revenge of Zeeka: Horror Trilogy comprises the first three stories in the award-winning series Revenge of Zeeka.

2016 - Zeeka's Ghost: Revenge of Zeeka Book 4– Zeeka's Ghost haunts Steven.

2017 - Resurrection: Revenge of Zeeka Book 5– the sudden appearance of a stranger, bothers Steven.

2017 - Zeeka Chronicles: Revenge of Zeeka: This multi-award-winning science-fiction novel, set in the year 2036, and inspired by the recent scare of the zika virus, where zombies and robots take center stage, has won four awards.

SELF-HELP

2017 - How to Write for Success: Best Writing Advice I Received – a popular guide for new and aspiring authors.

2021 – How to Write for Success: Volume Two. The book focuses on publishing and marketing.

POETRY ANTHOLOGIES

2019 – A Spark of Hope 1 co-authored by 49 authors, is a No 1 bestseller in Poetry Anthologies for prevention of suicide.

2020 - A Spark of Hope 2 coauthored by 64 authors, is also a No 1 bestseller in Poetry Anthologies for prevention of suicide.

2020 –Break the Silence coauthored by 84 authors, is a No 1 bestseller in Poetry Anthologies against domestic violence.

2021- Break the Silence: Volume Two coauthored by 91 authors is a No 1 bestseller in Poetry Anthologies, Inspirational and Religious Poetry, and a No 1 Hot new release.

2022- Peace Begins with Us – Poetic verses on Love, Peace and Humanity by members of HTWFSLN.

MAGAZINES

March 2021 - How to Write for Success Literary Magazine: Anniversary Issue. A No 1 bestseller.

Sept 2021- How to Write for Success: Literary magazine - Second Issue.

February 2022 – How to Write for Success Literary Magazine – Third Issue.

HE IS THE ONE

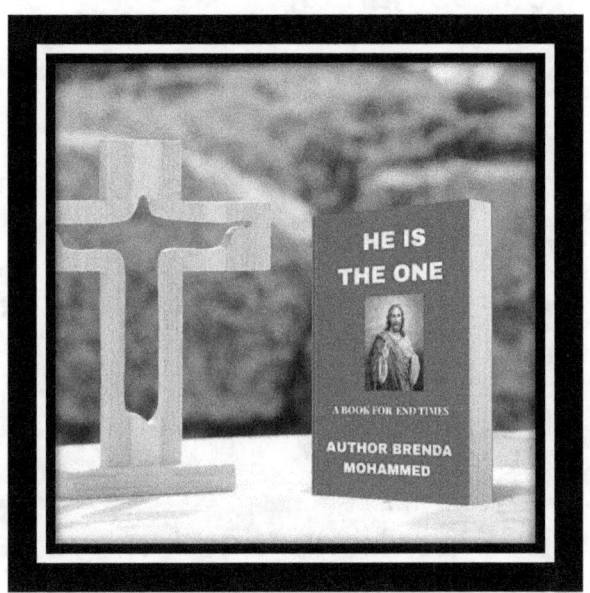

Almost six thousand years, humankind has spent,

Discovering God's work, using scientific experiments.

God took only six days to create the world spheres.

To us, one day's work for Him seems like a thousand years.

To work miracles, God just has to lift his hands.

Answers billions of prayers daily to satisfy our demands.

Can we really understand the depth of his love?

The Omnipotent, Omniscient, and Omnipresent God above.

HE can remove every burden in your life.

HE does not want his children to live with strife.

HE is the Alpha, and Omega, is the Beginning and the End.

The impossible HE makes possible; HE is your Best Friend.

Turn to Him for all your needs, you'll never be alone.

When humans disappoint you, remember you're HIS own.

HE is the specialist in love matters, the great physician.

His love is unfailing and true, and HE is our salvation.

.

CHOSEN BY THE CREATOR

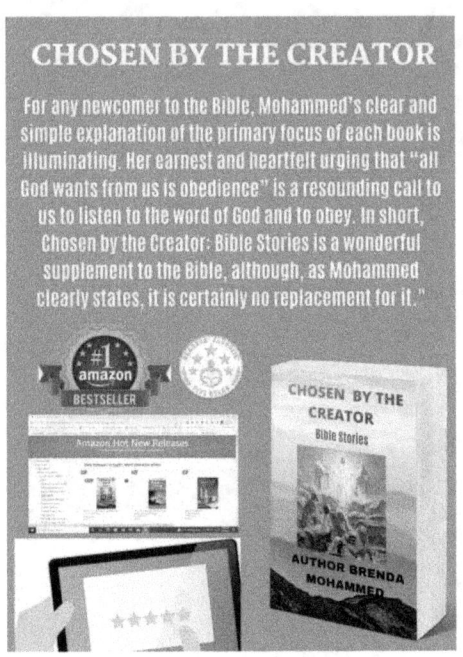

"Reviewed By Lois Henderson for Readers' Favorite

Chosen by the Creator: Bible Stories by Brenda Mohammed is aimed at helping the reader trace the line of descendants as far back as to the beginning of mankind, with the story of

Adam and Eve. Mohammed, who is a firm believer in the fact that "the Bible is God's biography written by his chosen ones," explains, with the help of quotations from the Bible, how the contents of each of its books relate to the whole.

Mohammed ends Chosen by the Creator: Bible Stories with additional material that provides true value for the reader, including the importance of having our names written down in the Book of Life; the text of her favorite two Psalms, 23 and 121 (which is my favorite, too) and a conclusion, confirming her desire (which she has successfully fulfilled) to write a story of God's chosen ones from each book in both the Old and the New Testament.

I love the way Brenda Mohammed, in her work Chosen by the Creator: Bible Stories, affirms her desire that the stories she retells in accessible and straightforward language will convince the reader of the genuineness and authenticity of their source in divine will.

For any newcomer to the Bible, Mohammed's clear and simple explanation of the primary focus of each book is illuminating.

Her earnest and heartfelt urging that "all God wants from us is obedience" is a resounding call to us to listen to the word of God and to obey.

In short, Chosen by the Creator: Bible Stories is a wonderful supplement to the Bible, although, as Mohammed clearly states, it is certainly no replacement for it."

COPYRIGHT